JOINT PAIN

RELIEF

A Guide to Natural Treatments and Self-Care Strategies

Eckman Johnson

TABLE OF CONTENTS

INTRODUCTION..4

What exactly is Joint Pain? 6

CHAPTER 1..7

Understanding Joint Pain.................................7

Joint pain causes..9

Different types of joint pain.........................11

Risk elements...13

CHAPTER 2..16

Natural Joint Pain Treatments 16

Herbs and supplements 17

Acupuncture 20

Chiropractic treatment 22

physical therapy..24

CHAPTER 3..26

Self-Care Strategies for Joint Pain Relief...........26

Physical exercise and activity....................26

Diet and nutrition 28

Stress control 30

Sleep and relaxation 32

CHAPTER 4..35

When Is it Time to Seek Medical Help for Joint Pain? 35

Symptoms of severe joint pain 36

Conditions that may necessitate medical attention for joint pain 38

CHAPTER 6...**40**

People's success stories about using natural treatments and self-care strategies to manage joint pain. 40

Common questions and concerns about natural joint pain relief treatments and self-care strategies. 44

Answers to frequently asked questions about joint pain and its treatment...45

CONCLUSION **50**

The significance of a multifaceted approach to joint pain relief 51

Tips for maintaining long-term joint health....................................52

INTRODUCTION

John had been suffering from joint pain for many years. It began as minor aches and gradually progressed to a constant ache that prevented him from doing things he wanted to do. He tried over-the-counter medications and even went to the doctor a few times, but nothing worked. He was starting to get desperate.

John came across an article about natural treatments for joint pain relief one day. He became interested and decided to conduct some research. He discovered the significance of eating a healthy diet, getting enough exercise, and taking anti-inflammatory supplements. He also learned about herbal remedies and self-care techniques such as massage and heat and cold therapy.

John began to make some lifestyle changes. He started eating a healthier diet that included anti-inflammatory foods. He also began taking supplements and incorporating gentle exercise into his daily routine.

He noticed that his joint pain was lessening after a few weeks.

Encouraged, John decided to implement some of the self-care techniques he had learned. He began to experiment with massage, heat, and cold therapies. He also began to ensure that he was getting enough rest and practicing stress-reduction techniques.

After a few months, John was astounded by the improvement in his joint pain. It had significantly decreased, and he was able to do things he had not been able to do previously. He was grateful for the natural treatments and self-care strategies that had helped him find relief from joint pain.

John's experience is just one example of how natural treatments and self-care strategies can be used to find relief from joint pain. Continue reading to find out more about the causes and symptoms of joint pain, as well as natural treatments and self-care strategies that can help.

What exactly is Joint Pain?

Joint pain is a symptom of an underlying medical condition or injury that affects the joints as well as the surrounding muscles and tissues. It is caused by a variety of conditions, including arthritis, bursitis, tendinitis, gout, and other musculoskeletal disorders. Joint pain can range from mild to severe, and it can affect a single joint or multiple joints. Depending on the underlying cause, treatment options vary.

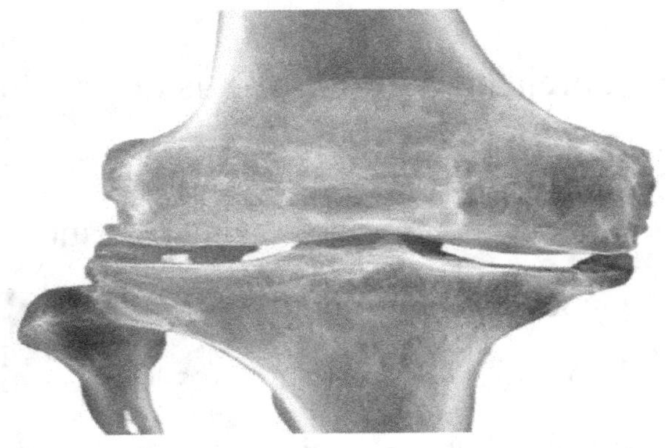

CHAPTER 1

Understanding Joint Pain

Joint pain is a common complaint among people of all ages, and it can be caused by a number of conditions, including arthritis, injury, infection, and autoimmune disorders. Joint pain affects nearly one in every two people, with the hips, knees, ankles, and elbows being the most common locations. Joint pain can be mild to severe, limiting a person's mobility and quality of life.

The first step in comprehending joint pain is determining the underlying cause. Arthritis is a leading cause of joint pain. There are numerous types of arthritis, such as osteoarthritis (OA) and rheumatoid arthritis (RA). The breakdown of cartilage in the joints causes OA, which causes swelling and pain. RA is an autoimmune disorder that causes inflammation of the joints. Injuries, such as a sprained knee or torn ligament, infection, such as gout or septic arthritis, and other medical conditions, such as fibromyalgia or lupus, can also cause joint pain.

Once the source of joint pain has been identified, doctors can devise a treatment plan to alleviate pain and improve mobility. Medication, physical or occupational therapy, or surgery may all be part of a treatment plan. NSAIDs (nonsteroidal anti-inflammatory drugs) are commonly used to treat pain and inflammation. Strength, flexibility, and range of motion can all be improved with physical and occupational therapy. Surgery may be required in more severe cases to repair damaged tissue or replace a joint.

Joint pain can be incapacitating, impairing a person's ability to work, exercise, and enjoy life. If joint pain persists or interferes with daily activities, it is critical to seek medical attention. Joint pain can be managed and improved with the right diagnosis and treatment plan.

Understanding joint pain is essential for correctly diagnosing and treating the underlying condition. Knowing what is causing joint pain can assist doctors in developing the best treatment plan to reduce pain and improve mobility.

People can better advocate for themselves and find the care and treatment they require if they understand joint pain and its causes.

Joint pain causes

Many conditions can cause joint pain, including injury, infection, arthritis, bursitis, gout, and others. A joint injury can cause pain, swelling, stiffness, and decreased mobility. Arthritis is the most common cause of joint pain in older people. It is caused by joint inflammation, which can be caused by wear and tear, an autoimmune response, or infection. Bursitis is an inflammation of the bursa, a fluid-filled sac that acts as a cushion between the joint and the skin. Repetitive motions, such as kneeling or squatting, are the most common cause. Gout is a type of arthritis caused by uric acid buildup in the joint, which can cause redness, swelling, and severe pain.

Joint pain can also be caused by infections. Bacterial infections, such as septic arthritis, and viral infections, such as the flu, are examples of these. Other diseases that can cause joint pain include lupus, Lyme disease, and rheumatoid arthritis. Additionally, as a side effect, certain medications and supplements can cause joint pain.

Overuse or strain can also cause joint pain. Sports-related repetitive motions can cause the joint to become inflamed and painful. Obesity and being overweight can also cause joint pain because the extra weight puts strain on the joint. Finally, some medical conditions, such as lymphedema, can cause joint pain by increasing joint pressure.

Joint pain is a common complaint, but it is treatable with the right medication. Depending on the cause of the joint pain, treatment options may include medications, physical therapy, lifestyle changes, or surgery. It is critical to consult with your doctor about the best treatment plan for you.

Whether caused by an injury, infection, arthritis, or another condition, joint pain can be incapacitating and interfere with daily activities. If you are experiencing joint pain, you should consult your doctor to determine the cause and receive the appropriate treatment.

Different types of joint pain

Joint pain is a common symptom of many diseases and conditions, and it can affect any joint in the body. Joint pain can range from a gentle ache to a sharp, burning sensation. Injury, arthritis, bursitis, gout, and a variety of other medical conditions can all cause joint pain.

1. Osteoarthritis: The most common type of joint pain, affecting millions of people, is osteoarthritis. When the cartilage that cushions the joints wears away, osteoarthritis develops. This can cause the bones to rub together, causing pain and stiffness.

2. Rheumatoid Arthritis: Rheumatoid arthritis is an autoimmune disorder characterized by joint inflammation and pain. It affects the joint lining, causing swelling, pain, and stiffness.

3. Bursitis is an inflammation of the bursae, which are fluid-filled sacs near the joints. It may result in pain, tenderness, and swelling.

4. Gout: Gout is a type of arthritis caused by uric acid buildup in the joints. It is distinguished by sudden, severe pain and swelling attacks.

5. Tendinitis: Tendinitis is an inflammation of the tendons, which connect muscles to bones. It is known to cause pain and swelling in the shoulders, elbows, wrists, and knees.

6. Fibromyalgia: Fibromyalgia is a chronic pain syndrome that causes widespread pain, fatigue, and joint and muscle tenderness.

7. Lyme Disease: Lyme disease is caused by the bacterium Borrelia burgdorferi. It can cause joint pain, swelling, and other symptoms.

Risk elements

Joint pain is a common condition that affects a large number of people. It can be caused by a number of factors, including age, injury, and medical conditions. A person's risk of developing joint pain can be increased by a number of risk factors.

One of the most common risk factors for joint pain is age. As people age, the cartilage in their joints wears away, causing stiffness and pain. Other age-related conditions that can cause joint pain include osteoarthritis and rheumatoid arthritis.

Another risk factor for joint pain is injury. Joint pain can be caused by joint trauma, such as a car accident or a fall. In some cases, the joint is permanently damaged, resulting in chronic pain.

Joint pain can also be exacerbated by medical conditions. Gout, lupus, and bursitis are all conditions that can cause joint pain. An underlying medical condition, such as diabetes or obesity, can also increase the risk of joint pain in some cases.

Certain lifestyle choices can also increase the likelihood of joint pain. People who are overweight, engage in high-impact activities, or perform repetitive motions may experience joint pain. Poor posture and a lack of exercise can also increase joint strain.

Joint pain can be incapacitating and have a negative impact on a person's quality of life. If you are at risk for joint pain, it is critical that you take precautions. Maintaining a healthy weight, exercising regularly, and practicing good posture can all help to reduce the risk of joint pain. If you are experiencing joint pain, you should consult with your doctor to determine the underlying cause and the best treatment options.

There are numerous causes and risk factors for joint pain. Knowing the risk factors can help you take precautions and treat any joint pain you may be experiencing.

Knowing the risk factors for joint pain allows you to take steps to lower your risk and manage any joint pain you may be experiencing.

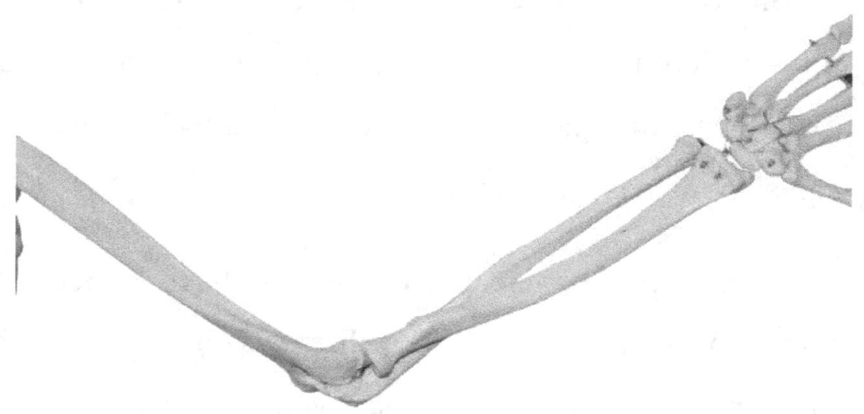

CHAPTER 2

Natural Joint Pain Treatments

Joint pain is a widespread issue that affects millions of people worldwide. While prescription medications are frequently used to treat joint pain, natural treatments can be equally effective and may be preferred by some people. Lifestyle changes, exercise, supplements, and herbal remedies can all be used as natural treatments for joint pain.

Changes in lifestyle are an important part of treating joint pain. Changing your diet, posture, and activity level can help relieve joint pain and improve your overall health. Eating a well-balanced diet, getting enough sleep, and maintaining a healthy weight can all help to alleviate joint pain. Stretching, yoga, tai chi, and strength training are all exercises that can help increase flexibility, reduce joint stiffness, and strengthen muscles.

Herbs and supplements

Joint pain is a common symptom of a number of conditions, including arthritis, bursitis, tendonitis, and gout. Many people use herbs and supplements to relieve joint pain naturally. While there is no conclusive evidence that any one herb or supplement is a miracle cure for joint pain, many of them have been shown in clinical studies to provide relief.

Glucosamine and chondroitin are the most commonly used herbs and supplements for joint pain. Glucosamine is a naturally occurring compound that aids in the formation and repair of cartilage, whereas chondroitin is a natural substance that aids in the maintenance of cartilage strength and flexibility. These two supplements, when taken together, can help alleviate the symptoms of arthritis and other joint conditions. Turmeric, ginger, Boswellia, bromelain, and cayenne pepper are some other herbs and supplements that are commonly used to treat joint pain.

Turmeric is a spice that has long been used as an anti-inflammatory. It contains the active ingredient curcumin, which can help reduce inflammation and alleviate arthritis symptoms. Turmeric has also been shown in studies to help reduce joint pain and stiffness.

Ginger is another herb that has been used to treat joint pain for centuries. It contains anti-inflammatory compounds that can aid in the reduction of swelling and pain. Ginger is also thought to aid in circulation and stiffness reduction.

Boswellia is a herb derived from the resin of an Indian tree. It contains anti-inflammatory compounds that can help arthritis patients reduce swelling and improve mobility. Boswellia has also been shown in studies to help reduce pain and stiffness in people suffering from osteoarthritis.

Bromelain is an anti-inflammatory digestive enzyme that is found in pineapple. It has been shown in studies to help reduce joint pain, swelling, and stiffness.

Cayenne pepper contains capsaicin, which is thought to reduce inflammation and pain in the joints. It can also help with joint stiffness and mobility.

Herbs and supplements can be a great addition to a healthy lifestyle and can help with joint pain relief. However, before taking any herbs or supplements, consult with your doctor because they may interact with certain medications. Furthermore, some herbs may not be suitable for certain people, such as pregnant women or those suffering from certain medical conditions.

Finally, herbs and supplements can be excellent options for people suffering from joint pain. While they are not a cure-all, they can help reduce inflammation, improve circulation, and alleviate pain and stiffness. However, before taking any herbs or supplements, consult with your doctor first because they can interact with certain medications and are not always safe for everyone.

Acupuncture

Acupuncture is a traditional Chinese medicine treatment that has been used for centuries to treat a wide range of ailments, including joint pain. It is based on the idea that the body's energy channels, or meridians, can be manipulated to improve health and well-being. Acupuncture stimulates specific points on the body, often with thin needles inserted into the skin. Endorphins, the body's natural pain relievers, are thought to be released when these points are stimulated.

Acupuncture has been shown to be effective in the treatment of joint pain, including arthritis and chronic musculoskeletal conditions. It can also aid in the reduction of inflammation, the improvement of blood circulation, and the reduction of stress. Acupuncture has been shown in studies to be more effective than traditional drugs in relieving joint pain, and it can even be used in conjunction with traditional treatments.

Acupuncture is usually used on a regular basis to treat joint pain, usually once or twice a week for a month or two. The acupuncturist will use thin needles to target specific areas of the body during the treatment. These needles are typically inserted into the skin and held there for 15 to 30 minutes. To stimulate the points further, the acupuncturist may use electrical stimulation, heat, or pressure.

Acupuncture is generally thought to be safe and is frequently used as an alternative to more invasive treatments like surgery. Before beginning treatment, it is critical to discuss all of the potential risks and benefits of acupuncture with your doctor. Furthermore, it is critical to locate an experienced acupuncturist who is trained in the specific type of treatment you seek.

Acupuncture can be a very effective and natural way to relieve joint pain and improve overall health.

However, it is critical to remember that it is not a replacement for traditional medical treatments and should always be used in conjunction with other forms of treatment.

If you're thinking about getting acupuncture for joint pain, talk to your doctor first. Your doctor may be able to refer you to a qualified acupuncturist or recommend alternative treatments that are more suitable for your condition.

Chiropractic treatment

Chiropractic care is a type of complementary medicine that is used to treat joint pain. It focuses on the diagnosis, treatment, and prevention of musculoskeletal disorders, as well as the effects of these disorders on the nervous system and overall health. It is a type of manual therapy that employs a hands-on approach to musculoskeletal and nervous system disorders diagnosis, treatment, and prevention.

Chiropractors treat joint pain with a variety of techniques, including spinal manipulation, massage, stretching, and exercise. They also apply pressure to the affected areas with special instruments. The treatment goal is to alleviate pain, restore joint mobility, and improve overall health.

Back pain, neck pain, headaches, sciatica, and sports injuries have all been shown to benefit from chiropractic care. It can also be used to treat joint pain issues such as arthritis and bursitis.

It is critical to seek treatment for joint pain from a qualified chiropractor. An experienced chiropractor can evaluate your situation and create a customized treatment plan to address the underlying cause of your joint pain. This treatment plan may include lifestyle modifications such as better posture, strengthening exercises, and dietary changes.

Chiropractic care can alleviate joint pain and improve overall health.

It is critical to seek the advice of a qualified chiropractor to ensure that you receive the best possible care. Joint pain can be managed and symptoms reduced or eliminated with proper treatment.

To summarize, chiropractic care is an effective method of treating joint pain. It is critical to seek the advice of a qualified chiropractor to ensure that you receive the best possible care. Joint pain can be managed and symptoms reduced or eliminated with proper treatment.

physical therapy

For people who suffer from joint pain, physical therapy is an effective treatment option. A number of conditions, including arthritis, bursitis, tendonitis, and gout, can cause joint pain. Physical therapy can help reduce inflammation, increase the range of motion, and strengthen and stretch muscles.

The physical therapist will evaluate the patient's condition and devise a customized treatment plan. This plan may include exercises to increase strength and flexibility, manual therapy to reduce pain and improve range of motion, and modalities to reduce inflammation such as ultrasound or electrical stimulation. To protect the joint, the therapist may also use taping, bracing, or other assistive devices.

Patients suffering from joint pain may be encouraged to do stretching and strengthening exercises at home in between physical therapy sessions. The goal is to alleviate pain while also improving the range of motion, strength, and function. Patients should avoid activities that aggravate their pain or cause further joint damage.

Joint pain can be effectively treated with physical therapy. Working with a physical therapist who can assess the patient's condition and develop an individualized treatment plan is essential. Patients can reduce pain and improve joint function with proper treatment.

CHAPTER 3

Self-Care Strategies for Joint Pain Relief

Self-care strategies are essential for dealing with joint pain. Many people experience joint pain as a result of arthritis, injury, or another cause. Creating a self-care plan can assist in relieving pain, reducing disability, and improving the overall quality of life.

Identifying the source of the pain is the first step in developing a self-care plan for joint pain. A physical examination, X-rays, or other tests may be used to accomplish this. Once the cause has been identified, the best course of action to relieve the pain must be determined.

There are several methods for dealing with joint pain:

Physical exercise and activity

Exercise and physical activity are excellent ways to manage joint pain and lower the risk of developing it in the future. Regular physical activity can help to strengthen the muscles surrounding the joint, relieving pressure on the joint itself. Exercise can also improve your range of motion and flexibility, lowering your risk of future joint problems.

Low-impact exercise is the best type of exercise for joint pain. This includes activities like walking, swimming, and cycling. These activities are ideal for people suffering from joint pain because they are low-impact and help to reduce stress on the joints.

Strength training exercises can also help people with joint pain. These exercises are intended to strengthen the muscles surrounding the joint, thereby relieving pressure on the joint itself. This can lessen the amount of pain felt. Strength training can also help you improve your balance, lowering your risk of falling and further joint damage.

If you have joint pain, you should consult your doctor before beginning any new exercise routine.

Your doctor may be able to recommend exercises that are specific to your needs. Furthermore, your doctor may refer you to a physical therapist who can provide you with additional information and assist you in developing a personalized exercise plan tailored to your specific needs.

Diet and nutrition

Joint pain is a common issue that affects millions of people, and it can be caused by a number of factors such as age, injury, and medical conditions. Diet and nutrition are important in the management of joint pain because they provide essential nutrients and anti-inflammatory compounds that help reduce pain and inflammation.

A healthy diet rich in fruits, vegetables, whole grains, lean proteins, and healthy fats can help reduce inflammation and provide essential nutrients for joint health. Omega-3 fatty acids, which are found in fatty fish such as salmon and tuna, can aid in the reduction of inflammation and pain. Flaxseeds, walnuts, and chia seeds are also high in omega-3s. Many vegetables, including kale, spinach, and broccoli, contain antioxidants and anti-inflammatory compounds that can aid in the relief of joint pain.

In addition to a well-balanced diet, certain supplements can help with joint pain. Pain and inflammation can be reduced by taking glucosamine and chondroitin sulfate. Vitamin D, which is found in fortified dairy products and fatty fish, can also aid in the relief of joint pain. Turmeric and ginger, which are both available as supplements, have also been shown to be effective at reducing pain and inflammation.

Finally, it is critical to stay hydrated. Water lubricates the joints and reduces inflammation. Staying hydrated can also help with pain relief.

It is possible to reduce joint pain and improve overall joint health by eating a healthy diet and taking certain supplements.

Eating a well-balanced diet, staying hydrated, and taking certain supplements can all help to relieve joint pain.

Stress control

Joint pain is a common complaint that can be caused by a number of factors such as arthritis, injury, or overuse. It can range from minor and short-term to severe and long-term. Joint pain, regardless of the cause, can be a debilitating condition that interferes with daily life. Fortunately, there are several methods for dealing with joint pain, including stress reduction.

Stress management is critical in the treatment and management of joint pain. Stress can cause and exacerbate joint pain by causing the body to produce hormones such as cortisol and adrenaline, which can cause inflammation and muscle tension. Stress can also lead to other unhealthy behaviors, such as poor diet or a lack of exercise, which can aggravate joint pain.

Stress management can assist in reducing the impact of stress on joint pain. Relaxation, mindfulness, and cognitive behavioral therapy are all stress management techniques. Deep breathing, progressive muscle relaxation, and guided imagery are all relaxation techniques that can help reduce the body's physical response to stress. Mindfulness focuses on being present at the moment and can help to reduce stress. Cognitive behavioral therapy assists in identifying and addressing unhealthy thought patterns and behaviors that can exacerbate joint pain.

Aside from stress management, other safe joint pain treatments include exercise, physical therapy, and lifestyle changes. Exercise can help to strengthen and stretch the muscles around the joints. Physical therapy can assist in reducing pain, increasing range of motion, and improving overall joint health. Adhering to a healthy diet and maintaining a healthy weight can also help to alleviate joint pain.

Stress management is critical in the treatment of joint pain. It can help reduce the impact of stress on joint pain and can be used alongside other safe joint pain treatments. Joint pain can be effectively managed and improved with the right combination of stress management and other safe care.

Sleep and relaxation

Sleep and rest are essential components of safe joint pain treatment. When dealing with joint pain, it is critical to rest the affected joint in order to reduce inflammation and allow the body to heal. When the pain is severe, rest is critical to reducing the intensity of the pain and hastening the healing process.

Sleep is also required for the management of joint pain. Sleep is the body's natural healing mechanism, and it is required for the body to repair itself and relieve joint pain. People who do not get enough sleep are more likely to suffer from joint pain, according to research. Furthermore, sleep aids in the reduction of stress, which is a major contributor to joint pain.

When it comes to joint pain, it is critical to strike the right balance between sleep and activity. Excessive rest can cause stiffness and weakness in the affected joint, while insufficient rest can aggravate the pain. It is critical to get enough rest to allow the body to heal while also maintaining a healthy balance of activity.

In addition to sleep and rest, there are other safe joint pain treatment options. Stretching, massage and heat therapies can all help to alleviate joint pain. Over-the-counter pain relievers can also be used to treat joint pain. Before beginning any medication, consult with your doctor.

Sleep and rest are essential components of safe joint pain treatment. Sleeping and resting enough can help reduce joint pain and promote healing. Other therapies, such as stretches, massage, and heat therapy, can also help to alleviate pain and improve joint health. Before beginning any type of joint pain treatment, consult with your doctor.

Joint pain can be managed and healed with the right balance of sleep and activity.

When the pain is severe, it is critical to listen to your body and rest. Joint pain can be managed and healed with the right care and attention.

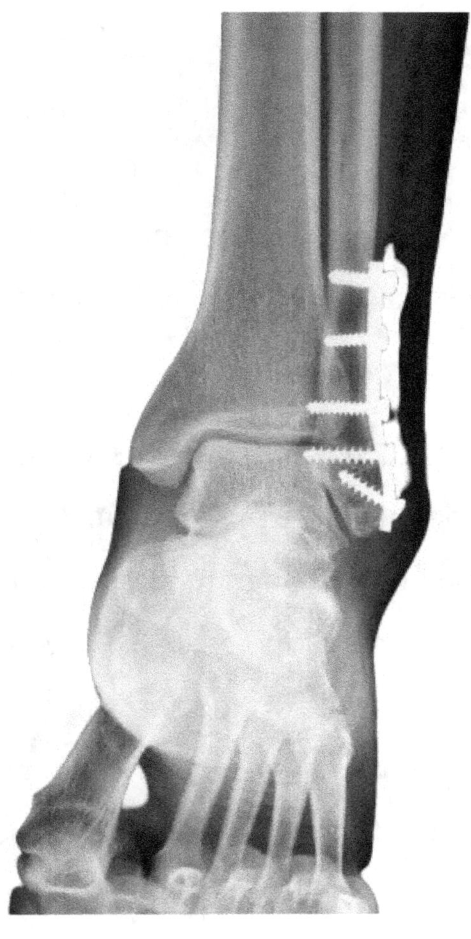

CHAPTER 4

When is it Time to Seek Medical Help for Joint Pain?

Joint pain can be caused by a variety of conditions, including arthritis, tendonitis, injury, and infection. Depending on the severity of the pain and other symptoms, seeking medical attention may be necessary at times.

If the joint pain is sudden and severe, seek medical attention as soon as possible. This is particularly true if the pain is accompanied by swelling, redness, warmth, or fever. These symptoms could indicate an infection or injury and should be evaluated by a doctor. Furthermore, if the joint pain is accompanied by other symptoms such as nausea, vomiting, or difficulty walking, seek medical attention immediately.

If the joint pain is chronic and lasts longer than a few days, it is critical to seek medical attention.

This is especially true if rest and over-the-counter medications are ineffective. A doctor can determine the source of the pain and recommend the best course of action.

Joint pain can be a sign of a serious medical condition such as rheumatoid arthritis, gout, or lupus in some cases. It is critical to seek medical attention if the pain persists or is accompanied by other symptoms such as extreme fatigue, weight loss, or fever.

It is important to remember that joint pain can indicate a variety of conditions, some of which necessitate medical attention. Seek medical attention if the pain is sudden, severe, or long-lasting. A doctor can determine the source of the pain and recommend the best course of action.

Symptoms of severe joint pain

A variety of conditions can cause severe joint pain, including arthritis, bursitis, gout, and tendonitis. An injury, such as a muscle strain or ligament sprain, can also cause it. Severe joint pain symptoms include intense pain and swelling in the joint, difficulty moving, stiffness, and redness. Warmth around the joint, a decreased range of motion, and grinding or clicking sensation when moving the joint are all possible symptoms.

The treatment for severe joint pain is determined by the underlying cause. Rest, ice, and elevation can be used to reduce swelling and pain if the pain is caused by an injury, such as a muscle strain or ligament sprain. To reduce inflammation and pain, nonsteroidal anti-inflammatory drugs (NSAIDs) such as ibuprofen or naproxen can be used. Physical therapy and surgery may be required in more severe cases to restore the full range of motion and strength.

Corticosteroids, DMARDs (disease-modifying antirheumatic drugs), and biologics may be prescribed to reduce inflammation and pain in cases of arthritis, bursitis, gout, or tendonitis. Physical therapy, heat and cold therapy, stretching, and massage are some other treatments that can be used to reduce pain and improve joint mobility.

Conditions that may necessitate medical attention for joint pain

Joint pain is a common complaint that can be caused by a number of different conditions. Joint pain may necessitate medical attention in some cases. These are some of the conditions:

Arthritis: Arthritis is a common cause of joint pain that can be caused by both wear and tear as well as an underlying autoimmune disorder. Treatment for arthritis may include medications, physical therapy, or even surgery, depending on the type.

Bursitis: Bursitis is an inflammation of the bursa, which is a small fluid-filled sac that cushions the joints. Corticosteroid injections or anti-inflammatory medications may be used to provide relief in some cases.

Tendinitis: Tendinitis is an inflammation of the tendons, which connect the muscles to the bones. Rest, ice, and nonsteroidal anti-inflammatory drugs are commonly used in treatment. Surgery may be required in severe cases.

Sprains and Strains: Sprains and strains are caused by ligament and muscle stretching or tearing. Rest, ice, and over-the-counter pain relievers are commonly used in treatment. In severe cases, surgery may be required.

Gout: Gout is a type of arthritis caused by an accumulation of uric acid crystals in the joints. Medications are typically used to reduce inflammation, pain, and uric acid levels.

Joint pain can be caused by an infection or another underlying medical condition in some cases. If self-care measures do not alleviate joint pain, it is critical to see a doctor for an evaluation.

CHAPTER 6

People's success stories about using natural treatments and self-care strategies to manage joint pain.

1. Sandra discovered the power of natural treatments after years of struggling with joint pain. She began a daily stretching, yoga poses, and meditation routine. Her joint pain had significantly decreased after a few weeks, and she was able to resume her active lifestyle.

2. Peter was told he would have to take medication for the rest of his life after being diagnosed with arthritis. Instead, he decided to experiment with natural treatments and self-care techniques. He was able to manage his joint pain without medication after a few months and could even run and hike on a regular basis.

3. Amanda found relief from chronic joint pain through natural treatments and self-care strategies after years of suffering. Massage, heat therapy, and specific exercises

became part of her daily routine. Her joint pain had subsided after a few months, and she was able to move more freely and without pain.

4. Jennifer was told to start taking medication after being diagnosed with rheumatoid arthritis. Instead, she decided to try natural treatments and self-care strategies. Her joint pain had significantly decreased after a few months, and she was able to resume a more active lifestyle.

5. After years of suffering from severe joint pain, John discovered natural treatments and self-care techniques. He began a daily stretching, yoga poses, and meditation routine. After a few weeks, his joint pain subsided significantly, and he was able to resume his active lifestyle.

6. Mark decided to try natural treatments and self-care strategies instead of medication after being diagnosed with gout. In his daily routine, he included massage, heat therapy, and specific exercises. After a few months, his

joint pain had significantly decreased, and he was able to resume a more active lifestyle.

7. Sarah discovered the power of natural treatments after years of struggling with joint pain. She began a daily stretching, yoga poses, and meditation routine. Her joint pain had significantly decreased after a few weeks, and she was able to resume an active lifestyle with minimal pain.

8. Steve found relief from natural treatments and self-care strategies after being diagnosed with osteoarthritis. In his daily routine, he included massage, heat therapy, and specific exercises. After a few months, his joint pain had subsided and he could move more freely and painlessly.

9. Sarah decided to try natural treatments and self-care strategies after years of suffering from chronic joint pain. Massage, heat therapy, and specific exercises became part of her daily routine. Her joint pain had subsided after

a few months, and she was able to move more freely and without pain.

10. Tom was told he would have to take medication for the rest of his life after being diagnosed with psoriatic arthritis. Instead, he decided to experiment with natural treatments and self-care techniques. He was able to manage his joint pain without medication after a few months and could even go for walks again.

These are just a few of the many success stories of people who have managed their joint pain with natural treatments and self-care strategies. If you are experiencing joint pain, don't be afraid to look into natural treatments and self-care strategies.

Common questions and concerns about natural joint pain relief treatments and self-care strategies.

1. How effective are natural joint pain relief treatments?

2. Are there any risks to using natural treatments?

3. Can natural treatments be used in conjunction with conventional treatments?

4. What self-care strategies can I employ to manage joint pain?

5. Is there any evidence to support the effectiveness of natural joint pain treatments?

6. Should I avoid any natural supplements or herbs if I have joint pain?

7. What lifestyle changes can I make to alleviate joint pain?

8. How quickly can I expect natural treatments to produce results?

9. What foods or activities can help alleviate joint pain?

10. What are the most effective natural treatments for various types of joint pain?

Answers to frequently asked questions about joint pain and its treatment.

1. Misconception: Arthritis is always the cause of joint pain.

Answer: A number of conditions, including arthritis, bursitis, tendinitis, and muscle strain, can cause joint pain. It is critical to consult with your doctor to determine the source of your joint pain so that a treatment plan can be tailored to your specific requirements.

2. Misconception: Pain medication is the only treatment option for joint pain.

Answer: While pain medication can help with joint pain, it is not the only option. Physical therapy, exercise, and lifestyle changes can all help to alleviate joint pain. Certain dietary supplements and topical creams may also help reduce inflammation and improve joint function.

3. Myth: Joint replacement surgery is the only option for treating severe joint pain.

Answer: Joint replacement surgery is an effective treatment option for severe joint pain, but it is not the only one. Injections, physical therapy, exercise, and lifestyle changes are some other treatments that can help reduce joint pain and improve joint function. It is critical to consult with your doctor to determine which treatment option is best for your specific situation.

4. Misconception: Joint pain is a natural part of the aging process.

Answer: Joint pain is not a normal part of aging and can be caused by a number of different conditions. It is critical to consult with your doctor in order to obtain an accurate diagnosis and develop a treatment plan that addresses the underlying cause of your joint pain.

5. Misconception: Joint pain is curable.

While joint pain can be managed and improved, it is not always curable. The treatment goal is to reduce pain and improve joint function. Because treatment plans are tailored to each individual, it is critical to consult with your doctor to determine the best course of action for your specific situation.

6. Misconception: The best way to treat joint pain is to rest.

Answer: While rest can help relieve joint pain in the short term, long-term relief requires more comprehensive treatment. Physical therapy, exercise, dietary changes, and certain medications can all help to alleviate joint pain and improve joint function. It is critical to consult with your doctor to determine the best treatment plan for your specific situation.

7. Misconception: Exercise aggravates joint pain.

Exercise can help to reduce joint pain and improve joint function. Swimming, yoga, and walking are low-impact activities that can help improve strength and flexibility without putting too much strain on the joints. Consult your doctor to determine the best type of exercise for you.

8. Myth: Joint pain is unimportant and should be ignored.

Answer: Joint pain is a symptom of a medical condition that should not be ignored. It is critical to consult with your doctor to determine the cause of your joint pain so that a treatment plan can be tailored to your specific requirements.

9. Myth: Taking supplements or vitamins will alleviate joint pain.

Answer: While supplements and vitamins can help with joint pain, they are not a cure. It is critical to consult with your doctor in order to determine the source of your joint pain and develop a treatment plan that addresses the underlying cause.

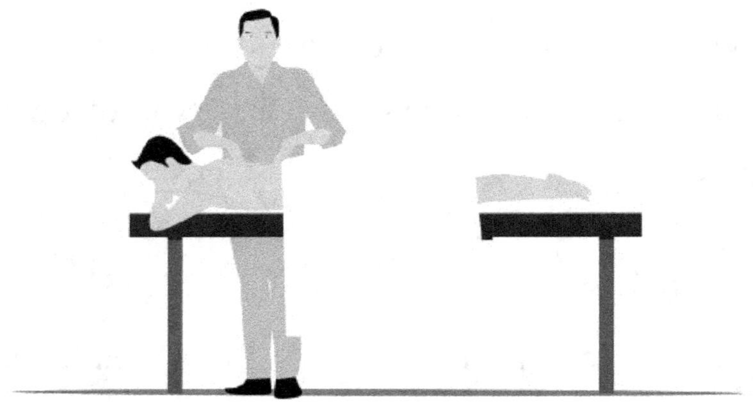

CONCLUSION

The natural treatments and self-care strategies discussed in this guide are safe and effective ways to manage joint pain. These treatments not only provide pain relief but also promote overall joint health. Joint pain can be managed and improved with a combination of lifestyle changes, dietary changes, and natural remedies. Individuals can take control of their joint pain and live a healthier, more active life with the right knowledge and dedication.

Living with joint pain can be a difficult and painful experience. Individuals can manage and reduce their pain with the right natural treatments and self-care strategies. Joint pain can be managed and improved with a combination of lifestyle changes, dietary changes, and natural remedies, allowing people to live healthier and more active lives.

As a result, the natural treatments and self-care strategies discussed in this guide offer an effective and risk-free method of managing joint pain. Individuals who follow these strategies can gain control of their joint pain and live healthier, more active and enjoyable life.

The significance of a multifaceted approach to joint pain relief

A holistic approach to joint pain relief is critical because it considers the entire person rather than just the physical symptoms of pain. This approach considers a person's lifestyle, environmental factors, emotional and mental health, and other factors that can contribute to joint pain. It also considers all possible treatments, such as lifestyle changes, physical therapy, medications, and alternative therapies.

A holistic approach aids in identifying the source of the pain and developing a treatment plan that addresses not only the physical symptoms but also any underlying causes. This approach can help reduce the risk of chronic pain as well as the need for medications. It is important to remember that a holistic approach does not always imply a natural approach; it simply means looking at all aspects of the person's life and attempting to identify any potential causes of pain.

The holistic approach can also be beneficial because it can help to improve overall well-being and reduce stress, both of which can have an effect on joint pain. This approach can also help to improve the quality of life for those who have chronic joint pain by reducing the amount of time spent dealing with pain and improving the overall quality of life. Finally, a holistic approach to joint pain relief is important because it aids in determining the source of the pain and developing a comprehensive treatment plan that considers all aspects of the person's life.

Tips for maintaining long-term joint health

1. Eat a Healthy Diet: A healthy diet rich in whole grains, fruits, vegetables, lean proteins, and low-fat dairy will help to maintain joint health over time. Anti-inflammatory foods, such as omega-3 fatty acids and

antioxidants, can help to reduce joint pain and inflammation. Processed and refined foods should be avoided because they can contribute to inflammation and joint pain.

2. Exercise on a regular basis: Exercise on a regular basis can help to strengthen the muscles around the joints and maintain joint health. Low-impact activities like walking, swimming, and cycling are especially good for joint health. Strengthening exercises can aid in the development of muscle, which in turn supports the joints.

3. Stay Hydrated: It is critical to drink plenty of water throughout the day to maintain joint health. Water lubricates joints and reduces friction, which can cause pain and inflammation. Staying hydrated also aids in the removal of toxins from the body, which can alleviate joint pain.

4. Avoid Injury: It is critical to avoid joint injury in order to maintain joint health. Wear appropriate safety equipment when participating in physical activities, and

lift weights with proper form. Stop the activity and seek medical attention if you experience joint pain.

5. Get Enough Rest: Adequate rest is essential for overall health, including joint health. The body, including the joints, repairs itself while we sleep. Get seven to eight hours of quality sleep per night.

6. Stress Management: Because stress can contribute to joint pain and inflammation, it is critical to managing it. Relaxation techniques, such as yoga or mindfulness meditation, can aid in stress reduction and joint health maintenance.

7. Lose Weight: Being overweight can put additional strain on the joints, resulting in pain and inflammation. Losing weight can help to maintain joint health in the long run by reducing the strain on the joints.

8. See a Doctor: Seeing a doctor on a regular basis can help detect joint problems early on and ensure they are addressed. Your doctor can also give you advice and recommendations on how to keep your joints healthy.

You can help to maintain joint health in the long run by following these tips. A healthy diet, regular exercise, staying hydrated, avoiding injury, getting enough rest, managing stress, losing weight, and visiting the doctor can all help to maintain joint health.